FIX YOUR HUNGER HABIT AND CRAVINGS

101 Practical Guide to Overcoming Hunger Habits, Quit Cravings, Stop binge eating and lose weight.

Valerie E. Walters

TABLE OF CONTENTS

Do you ever find yourself reaching for food, even when you know you're not hungry? Or do cravings seem to dictate your choices, leading you to indulge in foods you know aren't good for you? Are you tired of feeling powerless in the face of relentless cravings and insatiable hunger? Do you find yourself constantly battling the urge to indulge, only to be left feeling defeated and frustrated? If so, you're not alone. Many of us grapple with the challenge of managing our hunger habits and cravings, often feeling powerless in the face of their relentless pull. Studies show that cravings and hunger habits can significantly impact our health and well-being, yet many of us struggle to overcome them. But why is it that so many of us find ourselves trapped in this cycle of temptation and guilt? Is there a way to break free from the grip of cravings and take control of our eating habits once and for all?

In "Fix Your Hunger Habits and Cravings: A Comprehensive Guide to Transform Your Relationship with Food," a groundbreaking book designed to help you conquer your cravings and reclaim control of your health and happiness. Within the pages of this book, you'll embark on a transformative journey of self-discovery and empowerment, learning to understand the root causes of your cravings and developing the tools and strategies needed to overcome them.

Drawing on the latest research in nutrition, psychology, and behavior change, this book delves into the science behind cravings and hunger habits, unraveling the mysteries of our body's signals and exploring the psychological factors that drive our desire for certain foods. Through practical exercises and actionable advice, it guides you on a path towards creating a balanced, sustainable approach to eating that nourishes and satisfies your body and the mindset needed to make lasting changes to your eating habits.

But this book is more than just a collection of facts and figures – it's a roadmap for transformation, a blueprint for a healthier, happier you. By uncovering the hidden triggers and patterns that fuel your cravings, you'll gain a newfound sense of freedom and control, empowering you to make informed choices and live your best life.

So, if you're ready to break free from the cycle of cravings and hunger habits that have been holding you back, if you're ready to embrace a life of vitality, joy, and self-confidence, then "Fix Your Hunger Habits and Cravings" is the must-have guide you've been searching for. Say goodbye to guilt and frustration, and say hello to a future filled with health, happiness, and endless possibilities. *Your journey to transformation starts here.*

PART ONE

THE NATURE OF HUNGER HABITS AND CRAVINGS

Hunger habits and cravings form the intricate tapestry of our relationship with food, influencing not just what we eat, but also when and why. At their core, hunger habits encapsulate the tendency to eat even when satiated, driven by a complex interplay of physiological and psychological factors. Cravings, on the other hand, are the intense desires for specific foods, often high in sugar, fat, or salt, which can override rational decision-making and lead to indulgence.

Characterized by the persistent urge to eat beyond the body's caloric requirements, hunger habits often manifest as mindless snacking, emotional eating, or habitual overconsumption. Despite experiencing physical fullness, individuals may find themselves reaching for snacks out of boredom, stress, or simply out of habit. These habits can perpetuate a cycle of overeating, contributing to weight gain, poor metabolic health, and an unhealthy relationship with food.

The causes of hunger habits and cravings are multifaceted, encompassing both physiological and psychological factors. Physiologically, hormonal imbalances, such as dysregulation of ghrelin (the hunger hormone) and leptin (the satiety hormone), can disrupt appetite regulation, leading to persistent feelings of hunger despite adequate caloric intake. Moreover, fluctuations in blood sugar levels, triggered by consuming high-sugar or refined carbohydrate foods, can exacerbate cravings and perpetuate overeating behaviors.

Psychologically, hunger habits and cravings are often influenced by emotional states, environmental cues, and learned behaviors. Stress, boredom, loneliness, or anxiety can trigger cravings for comfort foods as a means of coping with negative emotions. Additionally, environmental factors such as the availability and accessibility of food, social norms, and cultural influences can shape eating behaviors and perpetuate unhealthy habits.

Types of Cravings
Physical Vs Emotional Hunger

Understanding the difference between physical and emotional hunger is crucial for developing a healthy relationship with food and making mindful eating choices. While both types of hunger involve the desire to eat, they stem from distinct sources and manifest in different ways.

Physical Hunger

Bodily Cues: Physical hunger is characterized by physiological sensations in the body, such as stomach growling, lightheadedness, or weakness. These cues signal the body's need for nourishment and energy to function optimally.

Gradual Onset: Physical hunger typically develops gradually over time as the body's energy reserves are depleted. It is often triggered by factors such as the passage of time since the last meal, low blood sugar levels, or increased energy expenditure.

Satiety: Physical hunger is satisfied by consuming a balanced meal or snack that provides the body with the nutrients and energy it needs. Once satiated, the hunger cues subside, and feelings of fullness and satisfaction are experienced.

Emotional Hunger

Triggered by Emotions: Emotional hunger, on the other hand, is driven by psychological factors rather than physiological need. It is often triggered by emotions such as stress, anxiety, boredom, loneliness, or sadness.

Sudden Onset: Unlike physical hunger, which develops gradually, emotional hunger can arise suddenly in response to emotional triggers or environmental cues. It may feel intense and urgent, leading to a strong desire to eat specific foods for comfort or distraction.

Unsatisfied by Food: Emotional hunger is often insatiable and cannot be satisfied by food alone. Eating in response to emotional cues may provide temporary relief from discomfort or distress, but it does not address the underlying emotional needs.

The complexity of hunger habits, particularly the tendency to eat when already full, and cravings lies in the intricate interplay of physiological, psychological, and behavioral factors. Physiologically, hormonal imbalances and metabolic dysregulation can disrupt the body's ability to accurately perceive hunger and satiety cues, leading to an insatiable appetite despite being physically full. Psychologically, cravings are often driven by emotional states, stress, and learned behaviors, compelling individuals to seek comfort or distraction through food, even when not truly hungry. Additionally, ingrained behavioral patterns and environmental cues play a significant role in perpetuating hunger habits, with habitual eating behaviors and environmental triggers overriding feelings of fullness. Untangling this complexity requires a multifaceted approach that addresses both the underlying physiological imbalances and the psychological and behavioral factors driving cravings and hunger habits, empowering individuals to regain control over their eating behaviors and cultivate a healthier relationship with food.

Physiological Factors:
Physiologically, hunger and satiety are regulated by a complex interplay of hormones, neurotransmitters, and metabolic processes. Ghrelin, often referred to as the "hunger hormone," signals hunger to the brain, while leptin, known as the "satiety hormone," communicates feelings of fullness.

However, disruptions in these hormonal signals, whether due to hormonal imbalances, erratic eating patterns, or metabolic dysregulation, can lead to an inability to accurately perceive hunger and satiety cues. This can result in a disconnect between physical fullness and the desire to continue eating, contributing to the phenomenon of eating when already satiated.

Behavioral Patterns:
Hunger habits, such as eating when already full, often stem from ingrained behavioral patterns and learned associations with food. Habitual eating behaviors, developed over time through repeated actions and reinforcement, can become deeply ingrained and automatic, leading individuals to eat in response to environmental cues or habitual

triggers, regardless of actual hunger levels. Breaking these ingrained habits requires conscious effort and reprogramming of behavioral responses to food cues.

Impact on Health and Well-being:
The complexity of cravings and hunger habits has profound implications for health and well-being. Chronic overeating, driven by cravings or habitual eating behaviors, can contribute to weight gain, obesity, metabolic disorders, and an increased risk of chronic diseases such as diabetes, cardiovascular disease, and certain cancers.

Understanding the psychological and physiological factors at play in hunger habits and cravings is essential for individuals striving to manage their eating behaviors effectively. These factors interact in complex ways, influencing our relationship with food and shaping our dietary choices.

Psychological Factors:
Psychologically, cravings and hunger habits are influenced by a myriad of factors, including emotional states, stress, boredom, and learned behaviors.

Emotional eating, in particular, is a common response to negative emotions, with individuals turning to food as a source of comfort or distraction from discomfort. Moreover, environmental cues, such as the sight or smell of appetizing foods, social settings, and cultural norms, can trigger cravings and override feelings of fullness, leading to overconsumption.

Emotional States: Emotions such as stress, boredom, loneliness, and anxiety can trigger cravings and drive overeating behaviors. Food often serves as a coping mechanism for managing negative emotions, providing temporary comfort or distraction.

Environmental Cues: Environmental factors, including the availability, accessibility, and palatability of food, as well as social and cultural norms surrounding eating, can influence hunger habits and cravings. The sight, smell, or presence of appetizing foods can trigger cravings and lead to impulsive eating behaviors.

Learned Behaviors: Habits and routines surrounding eating, as well as learned associations between certain foods and pleasurable experiences, can contribute to the development of hunger habits and cravings.

Common triggers and patterns of cravings are multifaceted and can vary widely among individuals, but certain themes and patterns often emerge that shed light on the underlying factors driving these intense desires for specific foods. Understanding these triggers can empower individuals to recognize and manage cravings more effectively, ultimately supporting healthier eating behaviors.

Emotional Triggers: Emotional states such as stress, anxiety, boredom, loneliness, or sadness are common triggers for cravings. Food often serves as a source of comfort or distraction from negative emotions, leading individuals to seek out specific foods that provide a sense of pleasure or satisfaction.

Environmental Cues: Environmental factors such as the sight, smell, or availability of food can trigger cravings. The presence of appetizing foods, food advertisements, or social gatherings centered around food can stimulate cravings and lead to impulsive eating behaviors.

Social Influences: Social and cultural factors also play a role in triggering cravings. Social gatherings, celebrations, and cultural traditions often involve the consumption of specific foods that are associated with pleasure or enjoyment, leading individuals to crave these foods in similar contexts.

Learned Behaviors: Learned associations between certain foods and pleasurable experiences can contribute to cravings. For example, if a particular food is repeatedly consumed in response to positive experiences or rewards, it can become strongly associated with feelings of pleasure and trigger cravings in similar situations.

Nutritional Deficiencies: Cravings may also be driven by underlying nutritional deficiencies or imbalances in the body. For example, cravings for certain foods high in sugar, fat, or salt may indicate a need for specific nutrients or energy sources that are lacking in the diet.

Habitual Patterns: Habitual eating behaviors and routines can also contribute to cravings. If certain foods are regularly consumed at specific times or in response to particular cues, such as watching TV or feeling bored, cravings for these foods may become ingrained over time.

By identifying common triggers and patterns of cravings, individuals can develop strategies to manage them more effectively. Practicing mindfulness, addressing emotional needs without relying on food, and creating a supportive food environment can help individuals navigate cravings and make healthier food choices that align with their goals for overall well-being

.

The impact of hormones and brain chemistry on appetite regulation is profound and multifaceted, influencing our eating behaviors and food preferences in complex ways. Several key hormones and neurotransmitters play pivotal roles in signaling hunger, satiety, and food reward, ultimately shaping our appetite and dietary choices.

Ghrelin: Often referred to as the "hunger hormone," ghrelin is produced primarily by the stomach and stimulates appetite. Ghrelin levels rise before meals and decline after eating, signaling hunger and prompting food intake. Ghrelin acts on the hypothalamus, a region of the brain involved in appetite regulation, to stimulate the release of neuropeptide Y (NPY), a potent appetite stimulant.

Leptin: Leptin, known as the "satiety hormone," is produced primarily by fat cells and acts on the hypothalamus to suppress appetite and regulate energy balance. Leptin levels increase with adipose tissue mass and serve as a signal of long-term energy stores. Individuals with leptin resistance, a condition characterized by reduced sensitivity to leptin's effects, may experience persistent hunger and overeating despite high leptin levels.

Insulin: Insulin, produced by the pancreas, plays a crucial role in glucose metabolism and energy storage. Insulin levels rise after meals in response to elevated blood sugar levels, promoting glucose uptake into cells and facilitating energy storage. Insulin also acts on the brain to inhibit appetite and reduce food intake.

Dopamine: Dopamine is a neurotransmitter involved in the brain's reward system and plays a key role in regulating food reward and motivation. Food cues, such as the sight or smell of appetizing foods, can trigger dopamine release in the brain, leading to feelings of pleasure and reinforcing food-seeking behaviors.

Serotonin: Serotonin, another neurotransmitter, is involved in mood regulation and appetite control. Low serotonin levels have been associated with increased appetite, carbohydrate cravings, and emotional eating. Selective serotonin reuptake inhibitors (SSRIs), a class of antidepressant medications, are thought to reduce appetite and food cravings by increasing serotonin levels in the brain.

The intricate interplay of hormones and neurotransmitters in the brain regulates appetite and energy balance, ensuring that our bodies receive the nutrients and energy they need to function optimally. Disruptions in these systems, whether due to hormonal imbalances, metabolic disorders, or environmental factors, can lead to dysregulated appetite, overeating, and weight gain. By understanding the role of hormones and brain chemistry in appetite regulation, researchers can develop targeted interventions to address obesity and related metabolic disorders and promote healthier eating behaviors.

Addressing hunger habits, particularly the tendency to eat when already full, and cravings is crucial for overall well-being, as these behaviors can have significant implications for physical health, mental well-being, and quality of life.

Physical Health: Chronic overeating, driven by hunger habits and cravings, can contribute to weight gain, obesity, and a host of related health issues, including cardiovascular disease, type 2 diabetes, hypertension, and metabolic syndrome. By addressing these behaviors, individuals can better manage their weight and reduce their risk of developing chronic diseases, leading to improved physical health and longevity.

Mental Well-being: Hunger habits and cravings can also impact mental health and emotional well-being. Emotional eating, in particular, is often used as a coping mechanism for managing stress, anxiety, or other negative emotions. However, relying on food for emotional comfort can lead to a cycle of guilt, shame, and worsening emotional distress. By addressing these maladaptive coping strategies and developing healthier ways to manage emotions, individuals can support their mental health and cultivate greater emotional resilience.

Quality of Life: Hunger habits and cravings can detract from overall quality of life by contributing to feelings of guilt, shame, and loss of control around food. Individuals may experience reduced energy levels, impaired concentration, and decreased productivity as a result of fluctuating blood sugar levels and poor dietary choices. By addressing these behaviors and developing a healthier relationship with food, individuals can experience greater vitality, improved mood, and enhanced overall well-being.

Reflection Prompt

What do you already know about how the body signals hunger and regulates appetite? How does this knowledge influence your eating behaviors and choices?

How does your body typically signal that it's time to eat, such as stomach growling, feelings of emptiness, or changes in energy levels? How attuned are you to these cues, and how do you respond to them?

____

____

____

____

____

What emotions tend to accompany your cravings, such as stress, boredom, sadness, or happiness? How do these emotions influence your desire to eat, and how do you typically respond to them?

____

____

____

____

____

What stress management techniques do you currently use, and how effective are they in reducing stress-related cravings?

____

____

____

____

____

What types of foods and eating patterns help to keep your blood sugar levels stable and prevent fluctuations in hunger?

____

____

____

____

____

Do you notice any recurring behaviors or routines associated with cravings, such as late-night snacking, boredom eating, or mindless munching while watching TV? Consider how these patterns contribute to your overall eating habits and whether there are opportunities to make positive changes.

____

____

____

____

____

Are there specific nutrients or food components, such as sugar, salt, fat, or carbohydrates, that tend to trigger cravings? Consider how your body responds to different foods and whether there are healthier alternatives or substitutions to satisfy cravings.

____

____

____

____

How do you feel physically, mentally, and emotionally after indulging in cravings? Are there any negative effects on your energy levels, mood, or overall well-being?

____

____

____

____

What types of foods and eating patterns help to keep your blood sugar levels stable and prevent fluctuations in hunger?

____

____

____

____

Action plan

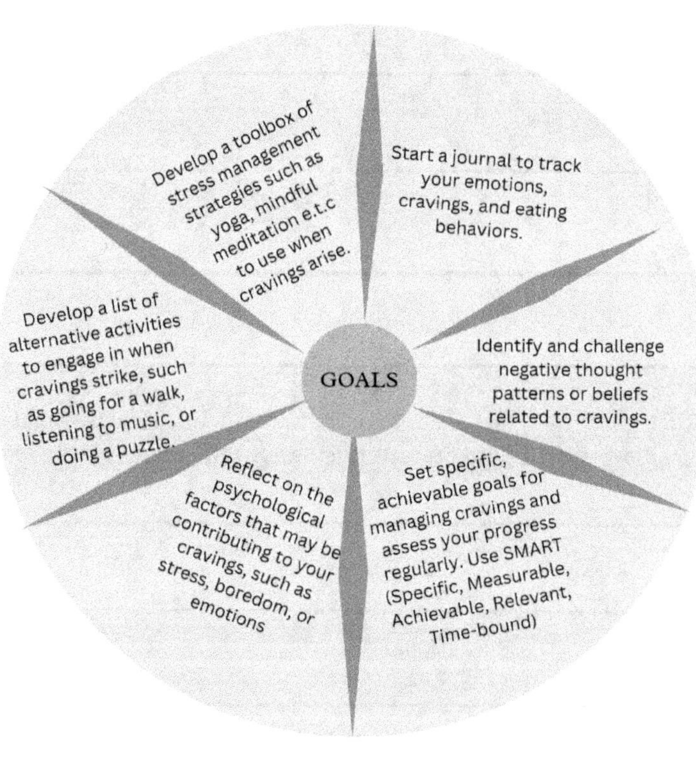

One step at a time let's go!

PART TWO

IDENTIFYING YOUR COMMON TRIGGERS AND PATTEN

Understanding and observing one's eating patterns is essential for cultivating a healthy relationship with food and making informed choices about dietary intake. Here's an exploration of eating patterns and how to identify and observe them:

Meal Timing: Pay attention to the timing of your meals throughout the day. Notice if you have regular meal times or if you tend to skip meals or eat irregularly. Observing your meal timing can help you identify patterns in your eating habits and establish a more consistent meal schedule.

Frequency of Eating: Consider how often you eat throughout the day. Notice if you tend to snack between meals or if you prefer to eat larger, less frequent meals. Observing the frequency of your eating can help you understand your hunger cues and energy needs.

Portion Sizes: Take note of the portion sizes of your meals and snacks. Notice if you tend to eat large portions or if you practice portion control. Observing your portion sizes can help you become more mindful of your food intake and prevent overeating.

Food Choices: Pay attention to the types of foods you typically consume. Notice if your diet is balanced and includes a variety of nutrient-rich foods, or if you tend to rely on processed or high-calorie foods. Observing your food choices can help you identify areas for improvement in your diet.

Emotional Eating: Be mindful of your eating behaviors in response to emotions. Notice if you tend to eat when you're stressed, bored, sad, or anxious. You can learn to recognize triggers and create more effective coping mechanisms by keeping an eye on your emotional eating habits.

Hunger and Fullness Cues: Tune into your body's hunger and fullness cues during meals and snacks. Notice if you eat when you're truly hungry or if you eat out of habit, boredom, or emotions. Observing your hunger and fullness cues can help you develop a more intuitive approach to eating.

To observe your eating patterns effectively, consider keeping a food diary or journal to track your meals, snacks, and emotions related to eating. Pay attention to patterns and trends in your eating behaviors, and reflect on how they impact your overall health and well-being. By becoming more aware of your eating patterns, you can make positive changes to support your health and nutrition goals

Triggers And Environmental Influences

Recognizing triggers and environmental influences on one's eating patterns, hunger habits, and cravings is essential for understanding the factors that drive food choices and behaviors. Here's an exploration of how to identify and recognize these influences:

Emotional Triggers: Pay attention to your emotional state and how it influences your eating behaviors. Notice if you tend to eat in response to stress, boredom, loneliness, sadness, or other emotions. Emotional triggers can vary from person to person and may manifest differently in different situations. Keep a journal to track your emotions and any patterns you notice in your eating habits.

Environmental Cues: Observe the environmental factors that influence your food choices and eating behaviors. This can include the availability and accessibility of food, social settings, cultural norms, and advertising. Notice if certain environments or situations trigger cravings or overeating episodes. For instance, certain foods or decadent eating habits may be connected to social events, festivities, or holidays.

Social Influences: Consider how the people around you influence your food choices and eating habits. Notice if you tend to eat differently when dining with friends, family, or coworkers. Peer pressure, social norms, and cultural traditions can all impact your eating patterns. Reflect on whether social interactions encourage or discourage healthy eating behaviors.

Routine and Habit: Identify any habitual behaviors or routines that are associated with cravings or overeating. Notice if you tend to snack at certain times of day or in specific locations. Pay attention to any patterns in your eating habits and consider how they may be influenced by your daily routine.

Cognitive Triggers: Become aware of the thoughts and beliefs that influence your food choices and eating behaviors. Notice if you have any automatic or habitual thoughts related to food, body image, or weight. Cognitive triggers can include beliefs about "good" and "bad" foods, dieting rules, or negative self-talk. Disprove any false or harmful ideas that lead to disordered eating habits.

Self-Reflection: Consider your eating habits and the circumstances that trigger cravings or episodes of overeating. Consider keeping a food diary or journal to track your eating habits, emotions, and environmental cues. Reflect on patterns and trends in your eating behaviors to identify potential triggers.

Situational Triggers: Determine which particular events or scenarios lead to periods of overeating or cravings.This can include times of day, such as late at night or after work, as well as certain activities or routines. Notice if you have any habitual behaviors or routines that are associated with food cravings or emotional eating.

To recognize triggers and environmental influences effectively, practice mindfulness and self-awareness in your daily life. Keep a journal to track your thoughts, emotions, and eating behaviors

Mindful eating is a practice that involves bringing full attention and awareness to the experience of eating, without judgment or distraction. It encourages present moment awareness, tuning into the body's hunger and fullness cues, and savoring each bite with all the senses. With an attitude of non-judgmental awareness, mindful eating allows for the observation of thoughts, feelings, and sensations without labeling them as good or bad. It involves fully engaging the senses in the eating experience, appreciating the colors, textures, smells, and flavors of food. Mindful eating extends beyond eating itself to include mindful choices about what, when, and how we eat, as well as the eating environment. Overall, mindful eating fosters a more conscious and intentional relationship with food, promoting healthier eating habits, improved digestion, and enhanced overall well-being.

Intuitive eating

Intuitive eating is a holistic approach to nourishing the body that emphasizes tuning into internal hunger and fullness cues, rather than relying on external rules or restrictions. By listening to the body's natural signals and honoring its needs, intuitive eating can help reduce hunger habits and cravings in several ways:

Honoring Hunger: Intuitive eating encourages individuals to recognize and respond to their body's signals of hunger. By honoring feelings of hunger rather than suppressing them, individuals can prevent excessive hunger that may lead to overeating or bingeing later on. Regular and balanced meals and snacks are encouraged to maintain stable energy levels and prevent intense hunger.

Respecting Fullness: Intuitive eating teaches individuals to pay attention to cues of fullness and satisfaction. By eating mindfully and stopping when comfortably full, individuals can avoid overeating and allow their bodies to regulate food intake naturally. Learning to recognize and respect the body's signals of fullness helps prevent the discomfort and guilt often associated with overeating.

Understanding Cravings: Intuitive eating encourages individuals to explore the underlying reasons behind food cravings. Rather than viewing cravings as mere signals for specific foods, intuitive eaters consider the emotional, physical, and situational factors that may contribute to cravings. By addressing these underlying factors and choosing satisfying foods in response to genuine hunger, individuals can reduce the intensity and frequency of cravings.

Embracing Food Flexibility: Intuitive eating promotes food flexibility and encourages individuals to give themselves unconditional permission to eat all foods. By removing the moralistic labels of "good" and "bad" foods, individuals can reduce feelings of deprivation and the subsequent desire to overindulge in forbidden foods. This food freedom allows for a more balanced and enjoyable approach to eating, reducing the likelihood of restrictive eating patterns that may lead to increased cravings.

Overall, intuitive eating fosters a compassionate and attuned relationship with food, helping individuals reduce hunger habits and cravings by trusting and respecting their body's innate wisdom. By listening to hunger cues, honoring fullness, understanding cravings, and embracing food flexibility, individuals can cultivate a sustainable and nourishing approach to eating that supports overall well-being.

Practicing Intuitive Eating

Practicing intuitive eating as a solution to hunger habits and cravings involves embracing a mindful and attuned approach to eating that honors the body's natural signals and cues. Here are some steps to implement intuitive eating:

Tune into Hunger Cues: Pay attention to your body's hunger signals and respond promptly when you begin to feel hungry. Eat regular meals and snacks throughout the day to maintain stable energy levels and prevent excessive hunger that may lead to overeating.

Eat Mindfully: Slow down and savor each bite of food, paying attention to the flavors, textures, and sensations. Avoid distractions such as electronic devices or television while eating, and focus on the experience of nourishing your body.

Stop When Satisfied: Listen to your body's signals of fullness and satisfaction, and stop eating when you feel comfortably satisfied. Avoid the urge to overeat or clean your plate out of habit, and trust that your body knows when it has had enough.

Explore Food Cravings: When you experience cravings, take a moment to explore the underlying reasons behind them. Consider whether the craving is driven by physical hunger, emotional needs, or environmental cues. Choose satisfying foods that address the root cause of the craving and leave you feeling nourished and satisfied.

Cultivate Food Flexibility: Give yourself permission to eat all foods without judgment or restriction. Allow yourself to enjoy a variety of foods in moderation, including those that may be considered indulgent or less nutritious. By removing the moralistic labels from food, you can reduce feelings of guilt or shame and develop a more balanced and sustainable approach to eating.

Practice Self-Compassion: Be kind to yourself and practice self-compassion throughout your intuitive eating journey. Accept that eating habits may fluctuate, and that it's normal to experience occasional cravings or overeating episodes. Approach each eating experience with curiosity, openness, and a willingness to learn from your body's cues.

By practicing intuitive eating, you can develop a healthier and more harmonious relationship with food, reduce hunger habits and cravings, and cultivate greater overall well-being. Trusting and respecting your body's innate wisdom is key to embracing intuitive eating as a sustainable and fulfilling approach to nourishment.

Mindful Eating Techniques

Practicing mindful eating techniques and strategies can be highly effective in avoiding hunger habits and cravings by fostering awareness, presence, and attunement to the body's natural signals. Here's how to incorporate mindful eating into your daily routine:

Eat Without Distractions: Create a calm and peaceful eating environment by eliminating distractions such as electronic devices, television, or reading materials. Focus solely on the act of eating and the sensory experience of the food.

Savor Each Bite: Take the time to truly savor and appreciate each bite of food. Notice the colors, textures, smells, and flavors of your meal. Chew slowly and mindfully, allowing yourself to fully experience the taste and enjoyment of the food.

Engage Your Senses: Engage all of your senses in the eating experience. Use your eyes to appreciate the presentation of the food, your nose to inhale the aroma, your hands to feel the texture, and your taste buds to savor the flavor. By fully engaging your senses, you can enhance your enjoyment of the meal and become more attuned to your body's hunger and fullness cues.

Listen to Your Body: Tune into your body's hunger and fullness cues throughout the meal. Pay attention to physical sensations such as stomach growling, feelings of emptiness, or subtle hunger pangs to determine when you genuinely need nourishment. Stop eating when you feel comfortably satisfied, rather than continuing to eat out of habit or in response to external cues.

Practice Gratitude: Cultivate an attitude of gratitude for the food you are about to eat. Take a moment to express gratitude for the nourishment it provides and the effort that went into preparing it. By approaching your meals with gratitude and appreciation, you can enhance your connection to the food and increase your satisfaction with the eating experience.

Stay Present: Stay present and focused on the present moment throughout the meal. If your mind starts to wander or you find yourself getting lost in thought, gently bring your attention back to the act of eating and the sensations in your body. By staying present and mindful, you can prevent mindless eating and reduce the likelihood of overeating or indulging in cravings.

Incorporating these mindful eating techniques and strategies into your daily routine can help you develop a healthier and more balanced relationship with food, avoid hunger habits and cravings, and promote overall well-being. By eating with awareness and presence, you can nourish your body, enhance your enjoyment of food, and cultivate a greater sense of mindfulness in all areas of your life.

Balancing nutrition is essential for correcting hunger habits and cravings, as it ensures that the body receives adequate nourishment to support overall health and well-being. Incorporating macronutrients—carbohydrates, proteins, and fats—in the right proportions is key to providing sustained energy, regulating appetite, and preventing cravings. Here's how each macronutrient contributes to addressing hunger habits and cravings:

Carbohydrates: Carbohydrates are the body's primary source of energy and play a crucial role in regulating blood sugar levels. Opting for complex carbohydrates such as whole grains, fruits, vegetables, and legumes provides a steady release of glucose into the bloodstream, helping to maintain stable energy levels and prevent sudden spikes and crashes in blood sugar that can trigger cravings for sugary foods.

Proteins: Protein is essential for muscle repair and growth, as well as for satiety and appetite control. Including adequate protein in meals and snacks helps to promote feelings of fullness and satisfaction, reducing the likelihood of overeating or experiencing hunger shortly after eating. Good sources of protein include lean meats, poultry, fish, eggs, dairy products, tofu, legumes, and nuts.

Fats: Healthy fats are important for supporting cell function, hormone production, and nutrient absorption, as well as for providing a sense of satiety and satisfaction after meals. Incorporating sources of unsaturated fats such as avocados, nuts, seeds, olive oil, and fatty fish helps to promote feelings of fullness and can help curb cravings for high-fat or processed foods.

In addition to macronutrients, understanding portion sizes and serving recommendations is crucial for maintaining a balanced diet and preventing overeating. Portion control helps to ensure that you're consuming the right amount of calories and nutrients to meet your body's needs without overindulging. Using tools such as measuring cups, food scales, or visual cues can help you gauge appropriate portion sizes and avoid consuming more than necessary.

Creating nutrient-dense meal plans that prioritize whole, minimally processed foods can further support balanced nutrition and help address hunger habits and cravings. Aim to include a variety of nutrient-rich foods from all food groups, including fruits, vegetables, whole grains, lean proteins, and healthy fats, in your meals and snacks. Planning meals ahead of time and incorporating a mix of flavors, textures, and colors can make eating nutritious foods more enjoyable and satisfying, reducing the likelihood of turning to unhealthy snacks or indulgences to satisfy cravings.

By incorporating macronutrients, understanding portion sizes, and creating nutrient-dense meal plans, you can effectively balance nutrition to correct hunger habits and cravings, promote satiety and satisfaction, and support overall health and well-being.

Role of Hydration in Curbing Cravings

The role of hydration in curbing cravings is often overlooked but immensely significant in managing hunger habits and cravings effectively. Here's an extensive exploration of how hydration can help individuals address cravings and foster healthier eating habits:

Appetite Suppression: Staying adequately hydrated can help suppress appetite and reduce cravings. Sometimes, feelings of thirst can be mistaken for hunger, leading individuals to reach for snacks or high-calorie foods when they're actually dehydrated. By drinking water throughout the day, individuals can prevent dehydration and better distinguish between true hunger and thirst, leading to more mindful eating choices.

Improved Satiety: Drinking water before or during meals can promote a sense of fullness and satisfaction, reducing the likelihood of overeating. Water adds volume to the stomach, which can help signal to the brain that the body is satiated, leading individuals to consume fewer calories overall. Additionally, choosing water-rich foods such as fruits and vegetables can further enhance feelings of satiety and help control cravings.

Regulation of Appetite Hormones: Adequate hydration plays a role in regulating appetite hormones such as ghrelin and leptin, which influence hunger and satiety signals in the body. Dehydration can disrupt the balance of these hormones, leading to increased feelings of hunger and a greater likelihood of experiencing cravings. By maintaining proper hydration levels, individuals can support optimal hormone function and better regulate appetite.

Energy Levels: Dehydration can lead to feelings of fatigue and low energy, which may trigger cravings for quick energy sources such as sugary snacks or caffeinated beverages. By staying hydrated, individuals can maintain optimal energy levels throughout the day, reducing the need for energy-boosting snacks and helping them make healthier food choices.

Supports Metabolism: Hydration is essential for proper metabolism, including the breakdown and utilization of nutrients from food. Dehydration can slow down metabolism and impair the body's ability to efficiently process nutrients, potentially leading to increased cravings for energy-dense foods. By drinking an adequate amount of water, individuals can support their metabolism and promote optimal nutrient absorption, reducing cravings for unhealthy foods.

Mood Regulation: Dehydration can negatively impact mood and cognitive function, potentially leading to increased stress or emotional eating. By staying hydrated, individuals can support cognitive function and mood stability, reducing the likelihood of turning to food for comfort or stress relief. Drinking water regularly throughout the day can help maintain mental clarity and emotional well-being, supporting healthier eating habits overall.

Craving Management Strategies: Incorporating hydration into craving management strategies can be an effective way to address cravings in the moment. When experiencing a craving, individuals can try drinking a glass of water first and waiting a few minutes to see if the craving subsides. Often, the body may be signaling thirst rather than true hunger, and hydration can help alleviate cravings naturally.

"Tips for Staying Hydrated Throughout the Day" is a helpful manual designed to assist people in sustaining optimal levels of hydration to promote general health and wellbeing, as well as efficiently managing cravings and eating patterns. This is a thorough analysis of methods for maintaining hydration:

Carry a Reusable Water Bottle: Keep a reusable water bottle with you throughout the day as a convenient reminder to drink water regularly. Opt for a bottle that is easy to refill and portable, allowing you to stay hydrated whether you're at work, school, or on the go.

Set Hydration Goals: Establish daily hydration goals based on your individual needs and lifestyle. Aim to drink a certain amount of water each day, taking into account factors such as age, weight, activity level, and climate. Tracking your water intake can help you stay accountable and ensure you're meeting your hydration needs.

Drink Water Before Meals: Make it a habit to drink a glass of water before each meal. Not only does this help hydrate your body, but it can also promote feelings of fullness and reduce the likelihood of overeating during meals. Additionally, starting each meal with water can help you make more mindful food choices.

Infuse Water with Flavor: Add natural flavor to your water by infusing it with fresh fruits, herbs, or vegetables. Experiment with combinations such as lemon and mint, cucumber and basil, or berries and citrus to enhance the taste of your water and make hydration more enjoyable.

Set Reminders: Use alarms, phone notifications, or hydration apps to remind yourself to drink water regularly throughout the day. Set reminders at intervals that work for you, such as every hour or with each meal and snack, to help you stay on track with your hydration goals.

Monitor Urine Color: One easy way to check your level of hydration is to observe the color of your pee.
Aim for pale yellow urine, which indicates adequate hydration, rather than dark yellow or amber, which may signal dehydration. Monitoring urine color can help you adjust your fluid intake as needed to maintain hydration.

Eat Hydrating Foods: Include foods high in water content in your diet, such as fruits and vegetables. Foods high in water, such as cucumbers, oranges, celery, and watermelon, help maintain general health and hydration while also offering vital minerals

Limit Dehydrating Beverages: Reduce consumption of dehydrating beverages such as caffeinated drinks, alcohol, and sugary sodas, which can increase fluid loss and contribute to dehydration. Instead, prioritize water as your primary beverage choice to support hydration.

Hydrate Before, During, and After Exercise: Drink water before, during, and after physical activity to replenish fluids lost through sweat and maintain hydration. Be proactive about hydrating before workouts, and continue to drink water regularly throughout exercise to prevent dehydration and support performance.

Listen to Your Body: Pay attention to thirst cues and listen to your body's signals for when you need to drink water. Thirst is a natural indicator of dehydration, so don't ignore it. Sip water slowly and consistently throughout the day to maintain hydration and support overall health and well-being.

By implementing these practical tips for staying hydrated throughout the day, individuals can support optimal hydration levels, reduce cravings, and promote healthier eating habits overall. Making hydration a priority as part of a balanced lifestyle can have a positive impact on overall health and well-being, helping individuals feel their best and thrive each day.

Reflection Prompt

What strategies do you currently use to cope with cravings, such as distraction techniques, mindful eating, or seeking support from others? How effective are these strategies in helping you manage cravings in the moment?

What times of day do you usually eat meals and snacks? Are there any consistent patterns or routines in your eating habits?

How do you typically react when you experience feelings of hunger or cravings? Do you tend to eat in response to these sensations, or do you try to resist them?

What specific foods or food groups do you find yourself craving most often? Are there any patterns or trends in the types of cravings you experience?

____

____

____

____

On a scale of 1 to 10, how intense are your feelings of hunger and cravings when they occur? How do these levels of intensity affect your ability to resist or manage them?

____

____

____

____

Discuss the different patterns of cravings you experience?

____

____

____

____

____

Think about your emotional state when you experience cravings: Do you notice a connection between your mood and your desire to eat?

____

____

____

____

Do you find yourself tempted by food advertisements, social gatherings, or peer pressure? How do these external factors affect your ability to make mindful choices about what you eat?

____

____

____

Who are the people in your life who support and encourage you in
your journey to fix hunger habits and cravings?

____

____

____

____

____

Take a moment to acknowledge and celebrate your successes, no
matter how small. What positive changes have you noticed in your
eating habits, and how do they make you feel?

____

____

____

____

Do you tend to eat larger portions than you need? How does portion size impact your feelings of fullness and satisfaction after a meal?

____

____

____

What strategies have you tried in the past to address your cravings and hunger habits? What worked well for you, and what challenges did you encounter?

____

____

____

____

____

Where are you when cravings typically occur, and what are you doing at the time? Are there any common factors or settings that seem to trigger cravings for you?

____

____

____

____

What times of day do you typically experience hunger or cravings? Are there specific triggers or situations that consistently lead to overeating?

____

____

____

____

Consider the types of foods you tend to crave; Are they typically sweet, salty, or savory?

____

____

Action plan

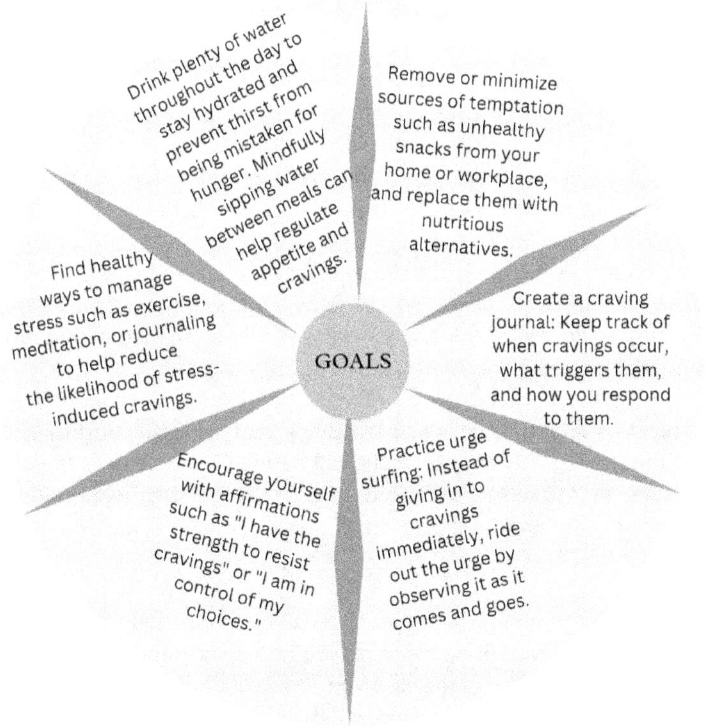

One step at a time let's go!

PART THREE

COPING WITH CRAVINGS

Managing cravings in the moment can be challenging, but with the right strategies, it's possible to navigate cravings effectively and make healthier choices. Here are some strategies for managing cravings in the moment:

Pause and Assess: When a craving strikes, take a moment to pause and assess the situation. Ask yourself if you're truly hungry or if the craving is driven by something else, such as boredom, stress, or emotions. By tuning into your body's signals, you can better understand the root cause of the craving and make a more mindful decision about how to respond.

Drink Water: Sometimes, thirst can masquerade as hunger or cravings. Before reaching for a snack, try drinking a glass of water and waiting a few minutes to see if the craving subsides. Staying hydrated can help reduce the intensity of cravings and keep hunger in check.

Distract Yourself: Engage in a distracting activity to shift your focus away from the craving. Take a short walk, call a friend, practice deep breathing exercises, or immerse yourself in a hobby or activity you enjoy. By redirecting your attention elsewhere, you can ride out the wave of the craving until it passes.

Practice Mindfulness: Mindfulness techniques can help you become more aware of your thoughts, feelings, and sensations in the present moment. When a craving arises, try practicing mindfulness by observing the craving without judgment or attachment. Notice the physical sensations associated with the craving and allow them to pass without acting on them impulsively.

Choose a Healthier Alternative: If you're craving a specific food, consider choosing a healthier alternative that satisfies the craving while still aligning with your nutritional goals.

For instance, choose a tiny serving of dark chocolate or a piece of fruit if you're desiring something sweet. Instead of reaching for chips when you're seeking something crunchy, try raw veggies or air-popped popcorn.

Plan Ahead: Anticipate cravings by planning ahead and having nutritious snacks readily available. Stock your kitchen with healthy options such as fresh fruit, nuts, yogurt, or cut-up vegetables. Having nutritious snacks on hand makes it easier to make healthier choices when cravings strike.

Practice Moderation: Rather than completely starving yourself, let yourself indulge in your favorite delicacies sometimes. Permitting periodic indulgences might lessen the chance of overindulging or bingeing on prohibited foods and help avoid feelings of deprivation.

Seek Support: Reach out to friends, family, or a support group for encouragement and accountability. Sharing your struggles with managing cravings can help you feel understood and supported, and receiving encouragement from others can help bolster your resolve to make healthier choices.

By incorporating these strategies into your routine, you can effectively manage cravings in the moment and make healthier choices that align with your nutritional goals and overall well-being. Remember that managing cravings is a skill that takes practice, so be patient with yourself and celebrate your successes along the way.

Coping with cravings and hunger habits often requires finding alternative activities and distracting techniques to shift focus away from food. Here's an extensive exploration of various strategies that can help:

Physical Activity: Engaging in physical activity can help distract from cravings and hunger habits by directing energy towards movement. Take a walk, go for a run, do a workout, or engage in a favorite sport or activity. Exercise not only occupies the mind but also releases endorphins, which can elevate mood and reduce cravings.

Mindfulness Practices: Mindfulness techniques, such as deep breathing, meditation, or yoga, can help bring awareness to the present moment and reduce the urge to eat in response to cravings. By practicing mindfulness, individuals can observe their thoughts and sensations without judgment, allowing cravings to pass without acting on them impulsively.

Creative Pursuits: Engaging in creative activities can provide an outlet for expression and distraction from cravings. Try painting, drawing, writing, crafting, or playing a musical instrument to channel energy into a productive and enjoyable endeavor.

Socializing: Spending time with friends, family, or loved ones can provide social support and distraction from cravings. Plan a get-together, have a phone conversation, or engage in a group activity to connect with others and shift focus away from food.

Learning Something New: Learning a new skill or hobby can help occupy the mind and distract from cravings. Take up a new language, enroll in a cooking class, learn to knit, or explore a topic of interest through online courses or books.

Outdoor Activities: Spending time outdoors in nature can have a calming and grounding effect, reducing stress and cravings. Take a hike, go for a bike ride, have a picnic, or simply sit and enjoy the sights and sounds of the natural world.

Self-Care Practices: Practicing self-care can help alleviate stress and reduce cravings triggered by emotions. Take a warm bath, pamper yourself with a massage or spa treatment, read a book, listen to music, or indulge in a favorite hobby.
Mindful Eating: Instead of giving in to cravings, practice mindful eating by savoring each bite and paying attention to sensations of hunger and fullness. Chew slowly, eat without distractions, and focus on the taste, texture, and aroma of the food.

Journaling: Writing down thoughts and feelings can help process emotions and reduce the urge to eat in response to cravings. Keep a journal to track cravings, identify triggers, and explore underlying emotions or patterns associated with food.

Volunteering: Giving back to others through volunteer work can provide a sense of purpose and fulfillment, distracting from cravings and promoting overall well-being. Volunteer at a local charity, community center, or animal shelter to engage in meaningful activities that benefit others.

By incorporating these distracting techniques and alternative activities into daily life, individuals can effectively cope with cravings and hunger habits, redirecting focus towards healthier and more fulfilling pursuits. It's important to experiment with different strategies to find what works best for each individual and to practice self-compassion along the journey towards balanced eating habits and overall well-being.

Developing resilience to cravings over time involves building mental strength, adopting healthy coping strategies, and creating sustainable habits that support long-term well-being. Here's how to stick with a resilient spirit without reverting back to old habits:

Understand Your Triggers: Identify the triggers that lead to cravings. These triggers could be emotional, environmental, social, or situational. By understanding what triggers your cravings, you can develop strategies to manage them more effectively.

Practice Mindfulness: Cultivate mindfulness by paying attention to your thoughts, feelings, and bodily sensations without judgment. When cravings arise, observe them with curiosity and compassion, rather than reacting impulsively. Mindfulness can help you create space between the craving and your response, giving you the opportunity to choose a healthier option.

Build Healthy Habits: Establish healthy habits that support your overall well-being. This includes eating a balanced diet, getting regular exercise, prioritizing sleep, managing stress, and nurturing supportive relationships. When your body is nourished and your needs are met, you'll be better equipped to resist cravings.

Develop Coping Strategies: Identify alternative coping strategies to deal with cravings when they arise. Try practices like deep breathing, yoga, meditation, writing, or partaking in enjoyable hobbies as an alternative to reaching for food when you're feeling down. Try out several tactics to see which one suits you the best.

Set Realistic Goals: Set achievable goals for managing cravings and celebrate your progress along the way. Break larger goals into smaller, manageable steps, and track your successes to stay motivated. Recognize that setbacks are a normal part of the process and use them as opportunities for learning and growth.

Build Resilience: Cultivate resilience by reframing setbacks as opportunities for growth and learning. Instead of viewing cravings as failures, see them as natural occurrences on the path to building healthier habits. Practice self-compassion and forgive yourself when you slip up, knowing that setbacks are a normal part of the process.

Practice Self-Compassion: Be kind and compassionate towards yourself, especially when you experience cravings or setbacks. Avoid self-criticism and negative self-talk, and instead, offer yourself words of encouragement and support. Show yourself the same compassion and consideration that you would extend to a friend going through a comparable situation.

Seek Support: Reach out to friends, family, or a support group for encouragement and accountability. Share your goals and challenges with others, and lean on them for support when you need it. Having a strong support network can help you stay motivated and resilient in the face of cravings.

Stay Persistent: Developing resilience takes time and effort, so stay persistent in your efforts to overcome cravings. Remember that change is a gradual process, and every small step you take towards managing cravings is a step in the right direction. Stay committed to your goals and believe in your ability to overcome challenges.

By incorporating these strategies into your daily life, you can develop resilience to cravings over time and stick with a resilient spirit without reverting back to old habits. With practice, perseverance, and self-awareness, you can cultivate a positive relationship with food and build a foundation for long-term health and well-being.

STRESS MANAGEMENT AND EMOTIONAL REGULATION

Stress management and emotional regulation are essential components of addressing hunger habits and cravings. By learning to effectively manage stress and regulate emotions, individuals can reduce the likelihood of turning to food as a coping mechanism. Here's how stress reduction techniques, emotional awareness, and healthy coping skills contribute to managing stress and emotions without relying on food:

Stress Reduction Techniques

Meditation: Meditation involves focusing the mind and redirecting thoughts to achieve a state of calmness and relaxation. Regular meditation practice can help reduce stress, lower cortisol levels, and promote emotional well-being.

Deep Breathing: Deep breathing exercises, such as diaphragmatic breathing or belly breathing, can activate the body's relaxation response, reducing feelings of stress and anxiety. Deep breathing helps calm the nervous system and promotes relaxation.

Yoga: Yoga combines physical postures, breathwork, and mindfulness to promote relaxation and reduce stress. Practicing yoga regularly can improve flexibility, strength, and balance, while also fostering emotional resilience and stress management skills.

Cultivating Emotional Awareness and Coping Skills

Emotional Awareness: Developing emotional awareness involves recognizing and understanding one's own emotions and their underlying causes. By becoming more aware of their emotions, individuals can better regulate them and make healthier choices in response.

Coping Skills: Building a toolkit of coping skills allows individuals to effectively manage stress and regulate emotions without turning to food. This may include strategies such as problem-solving, positive self-talk, seeking social support, engaging in enjoyable activities, or practicing relaxation techniques.

Healthy Ways to Manage Emotions Without Food

Mindful Eating: Practicing mindful eating involves paying attention to the sensory experience of eating without judgment. By tuning into hunger and fullness cues, individuals can develop a healthier relationship with food and reduce emotional eating.
Physical Activity: Engaging in regular physical activity can help reduce stress, elevate mood, and improve overall well-being. Whether it's going for a walk, jogging, cycling, or dancing, finding enjoyable ways to stay active can provide a natural outlet for managing emotions.
Creative Expression: Engaging in creative activities such as art, music, writing, or gardening can help channel emotions in a constructive way. Creative expression allows individuals to express themselves, process emotions, and find meaning and fulfillment outside of food.
By incorporating stress reduction techniques, cultivating emotional awareness, and finding healthy ways to manage emotions without food, individuals can develop resilience in the face of stress and cravings. Through consistent practice and self-awareness, it's possible to build healthier habits and cope with emotions in a positive and constructive manner.

Environmental Modifications for Success

Creating a supportive food environment at home and navigating food environments outside the home are crucial steps in maintaining healthy eating habits and managing cravings. Additionally, building a support network can provide accountability and encouragement, further enhancing success in addressing hunger habits and cravings. Here's how to implement strategies for each aspect:

Creating a Supportive Food Environment at Home:

Stock Up on Healthy Options: Fill your kitchen with nutritious, whole foods such as fruits, vegetables, lean proteins, whole grains, and healthy fats. Having healthy options readily available makes it easier to make nutritious choices and reduces the temptation to indulge in unhealthy snacks.

Minimize Temptations: Limit the presence of highly processed, sugary, and high-calorie foods in your home. Keep these items out of sight or in less accessible areas to reduce the likelihood of mindless snacking and impulsive eating.

Meal Planning and Preparation: Plan and prepare meals ahead of time to ensure you have balanced, nutritious options available throughout the week. Set aside time each week to plan meals, create shopping lists, and prepare healthy ingredients to streamline mealtime and minimize the need for unhealthy takeout or convenience foods.

Practice Portion Control: Use smaller plates, bowls, and serving utensils to help control portion sizes and prevent overeating. Pay attention to portion sizes and serve appropriate portions to avoid consuming excess calories.

Strategies for Navigating Food Environments Outside the Home:

Plan Ahead: Before heading out, anticipate potential food environments and plan accordingly. Bring healthy snacks or meals with you to avoid relying on unhealthy options when hunger strikes.
Make Informed Choices: When dining out or navigating food environments outside the home, choose options that align with your health goals. Look for menu items that are grilled, baked, steamed, or roasted, and opt for dishes with plenty of vegetables, lean proteins, and whole grains.

Practice Mindful Eating: Pay attention to hunger and fullness cues, and eat slowly to savor each bite. Avoid mindless eating or eating out of boredom, and tune into your body's signals to determine when you're truly hungry and when you're satisfied.

Building a Support Network:

Seek Accountability: Share your goals and challenges with friends, family, or a support group, and ask for their support and accountability. Having someone to check in with and hold you accountable can help keep you motivated and on track.

Find Encouragement: Surround yourself with supportive individuals who encourage and uplift you on your journey towards better health. Whether it's a workout buddy, a nutritionist, or a mentor, having someone in your corner who believes in you can make a significant difference in your success.

Join Supportive Communities: Consider joining online forums, social media groups, or local organizations focused on health and wellness. Connecting with like-minded individuals who share similar goals can provide valuable support, encouragement, and inspiration along the way.

By creating a supportive food environment at home, employing strategies for navigating food environments outside the home, and building a support network, individuals can empower themselves to make healthier choices, manage cravings, and achieve their health and wellness goals.

1. Meal prepping and batch cooking

Meal prepping and batch cooking are highly effective strategies for fixing hunger habits and cravings, providing convenience, consistency, and control over food choices. Here's how meal prepping and batch cooking contribute to addressing hunger habits and cravings:

Convenience and Time-Saving:
Meal prepping involves preparing meals or ingredients in advance, saving time during busy weekdays. By dedicating a few hours each week to meal prepping, individuals can streamline mealtime and avoid relying on unhealthy convenience foods or takeout options when hunger strikes.
Batch cooking allows individuals to prepare larger quantities of food at once, which can be portioned out and enjoyed throughout the week. Having pre-cooked meals or ingredients readily available reduces the need for cooking from scratch every day, making it easier to stick to healthy eating habits.

Consistency and Portion Control:
Meal prepping ensures consistency in meal choices and portion sizes, helping individuals maintain balanced and nutritious eating habits. By portioning out meals in advance, individuals can avoid overeating or reaching for unhealthy snacks when hunger strikes.
Batch cooking allows for portion control by pre-dividing meals into individual servings or containers. This prevents the temptation to overindulge and promotes mindful eating habits, as individuals can easily grab a pre-portioned meal when hunger strikes.

Healthier Food Choices:
Meal prepping and batch cooking empower individuals to make healthier food choices by planning and preparing meals ahead of time. By having nutritious meals readily available, individuals are less likely to rely on convenience foods or fast food options that are often high in calories, sugar, and unhealthy fats.
Batch cooking allows for the inclusion of a variety of nutrient-dense ingredients, such as lean proteins, whole grains, and plenty of vegetables.

2. Grocery Shopping Tips for Making Healthier Choices

Grocery shopping is a critical step in fixing hunger habits and cravings, as it sets the foundation for healthier eating habits at home. Here are some practical tips for making healthier choices while grocery shopping:

Plan Ahead:
Before heading to the grocery store, take some time to plan your meals for the week. Create a list of ingredients you'll need based on your planned recipes, ensuring you have everything you need to prepare balanced and nutritious meals.

Shop the Perimeter:
In most grocery stores, the perimeter is where you'll find fresh produce, lean proteins, dairy, and whole foods. Focus your shopping on the perimeter aisles, where the majority of nutrient-dense, minimally processed foods are located.

Fill Your Cart with Color:
Aim to fill your cart with a variety of colorful fruits and vegetables. Different colors indicate a variety of nutrients, so incorporating a rainbow of produce into your diet ensures you're getting a wide range of vitamins, minerals, and antioxidants.

Read Labels Carefully:
When selecting packaged foods, take the time to read labels and ingredients lists. Look for products with simple, recognizable ingredients and minimal added sugars, sodium, and unhealthy fats. Pay attention to serving sizes and nutrient content to make informed choices.

Choose Whole Grains:
Opt for whole grains such as brown rice, quinoa, oats, and whole wheat bread and pasta. Whole grains are higher in fiber and nutrients compared to refined grains, helping to keep you fuller for longer and stabilize blood sugar levels.

Prioritize Lean Proteins:
Choose lean sources of protein such as skinless poultry, fish, tofu, beans, lentils, and low-fat dairy products. Incorporating protein-rich foods into your meals helps to build and repair tissues, support muscle growth, and keep you feeling satisfied between meals.

Limit Processed Foods:
Minimize the amount of processed and packaged foods in your cart, as these often contain added sugars, unhealthy fats, and artificial additives. Instead, focus on whole, minimally processed foods that are closer to their natural state.

Stay Hydrated:
Don't forget to include beverages in your grocery shopping plan. Opt for water, herbal teas, and other low-calorie beverages to stay hydrated throughout the day. Limit sugary drinks, sodas, and energy drinks, which can contribute to cravings and fluctuations in energy levels.

Be Mindful of Portions:
Pay attention to portion sizes and avoid buying oversized packages or bulk items unless you plan to portion them out into smaller servings. Overeating can lead to feelings of discomfort and guilt, so aim to purchase foods in appropriate portions for your needs.

Stock Up on Healthy Snacks:
Choose nutrient-dense snacks such as fresh fruit, vegetables with hummus or Greek yogurt, nuts and seeds, whole grain crackers, or air-popped popcorn. Having healthy snacks on hand makes it easier to resist unhealthy temptations and manage cravings between meals.

By following these grocery shopping tips and making intentional choices about the foods you bring into your home, you can set yourself up for success in fixing hunger habits and cravings. By prioritizing nutrient-dense, whole foods and minimizing processed and unhealthy options, you'll nourish your body and support your overall health and well-being

3. Eating Out Strategies

Fixing hunger habits and cravings while dining out requires mindful decision-making and strategic planning. Here are some effective eating out strategies to help address hunger habits and cravings:

Research Menus in Advance:
Before heading to a restaurant, review the menu online to identify healthier options. Look for dishes that are grilled, steamed, or baked rather than fried, and prioritize meals rich in lean proteins, whole grains, and vegetables.

Opt for Lighter Preparations:
Choose dishes that are prepared using healthier cooking methods, such as grilling, roasting, or sautéing with minimal added fats. Avoid heavy sauces and creamy dressings, and opt for lighter alternatives like vinaigrettes or salsa.

Mindful Portion Control:
Be mindful of portion sizes, which tend to be larger in restaurants. Consider ordering appetizers or sharing entrees with dining companions to manage portion sizes and avoid overeating.

Load Up on Veggies:
Fill your plate with plenty of vegetables, either as sides or as the main component of your meal. Vegetables are low in calories and high in fiber, helping to promote feelings of fullness and satisfaction.

Watch Your Beverages:
Be mindful of liquid calories from sugary drinks, alcoholic beverages, and high-calorie cocktails. Opt for water, unsweetened tea, or sparkling water with a splash of lemon or lime to stay hydrated without consuming excess calories.

Customize Your Order:
Don't hesitate to ask for substitutions or modifications to suit your preferences and dietary needs. Requesting dressings on the side, swapping out fries for a side salad, or substituting whole grain options for refined carbohydrates can help make your meal healthier.

Practice Mindful Eating:

savor each bite slowy, paying attention to hunger and fullness cues. Avoid mindless eating and focus on enjoying the flavors and textures of your food to prevent overeating.

Stay Prepared for Cravings:
If you know you'll be tempted by unhealthy options, come prepared with healthier snacks or alternatives to satisfy cravings. Having a plan in place can help you make better choices in the moment.
Be Flexible and Forgiving:

Remember that eating out is meant to be enjoyable, and it's okay to indulge occasionally. If you do end up indulging in a less healthy option, practice self-compassion and move on rather than dwelling on feelings of guilt or regret.
By implementing these eating out strategies, you can make healthier choices while dining out and better manage hunger habits and cravings without sacrificing enjoyment or satisfaction.

Sleep and Rest

impact of sleep and rest on hunger hormones and cravings is profound, influencing appetite regulation and food intake in significant ways. Here's an exploration of how sleep and rest affect hunger hormones and cravings:

Ghrelin Regulation: Ghrelin, often referred to as the "hunger hormone," stimulates appetite and increases food intake. Adequate sleep and rest play a crucial role in regulating ghrelin levels. Research has shown that sleep deprivation can lead to elevated ghrelin levels, resulting in increased feelings of hunger and cravings for high-calorie foods. Conversely, getting enough sleep can help maintain ghrelin levels within a healthy range, reducing the likelihood of excessive hunger and overeating.

Leptin Production: Leptin is a hormone that signals satiety and regulates energy balance by suppressing appetite. Adequate sleep is essential for proper leptin production and signaling.

Sleep deprivation can disrupt leptin levels, leading to reduced leptin production and impaired signaling to the brain that the body is full. As a result, individuals may experience increased cravings and a tendency to overeat, even when they are not truly hungry.

Insulin Sensitivity: Sleep plays a crucial role in regulating insulin sensitivity, which is essential for glucose metabolism and energy balance. Poor sleep quality and insufficient rest can lead to decreased insulin sensitivity, increasing the risk of insulin resistance and metabolic disturbances. Dysregulated insulin levels can trigger cravings for sugary and high-carbohydrate foods, contributing to unhealthy eating habits and weight gain.

Cortisol Levels: Cortisol, often referred to as the "stress hormone," plays a role in appetite regulation and energy metabolism. Chronic stress and sleep deprivation can lead to dysregulated cortisol levels, which may increase cravings for comfort foods high in sugar and fat. Elevated cortisol levels can also disrupt hunger and satiety signals, leading to irregular eating patterns and poor food choices.

Brain Function: Adequate sleep is essential for optimal brain function, including areas of the brain responsible for food cravings and decision-making. Sleep deprivation can impair cognitive function and judgment, making it more difficult to resist cravings and make healthy food choices. Additionally, sleep deficiency can increase the reward value of unhealthy foods, leading to heightened cravings and a greater likelihood of overeating.

Benefits of Regular Physical Exercise in Reducing Cravings

Regular physical exercise and movement offer a myriad of benefits for overall health and well-being, including their role in reducing cravings. Here's how:

Stress Reduction: Exercise helps to reduce stress levels by triggering the release of endorphins, which are natural mood elevators. Many cravings, particularly those for comfort foods high in sugar or fat, are often triggered by stress or emotional factors. By reducing stress, exercise can help mitigate these triggers and reduce the intensity of cravings.

Improved Mood: Exercise has been shown to improve mood and alleviate symptoms of depression and anxiety. When mood is improved, individuals are less likely to turn to unhealthy foods or substances as a coping mechanism for negative emotions, reducing cravings for these items.

Regulation of Appetite Hormones: Physical activity can help regulate hormones that control appetite, such as ghrelin and leptin. Regular exercise can lead to decreased levels of ghrelin, the hormone that stimulates appetite, and increased levels of leptin, the hormone that signals fullness. This hormonal balance can help reduce cravings and promote healthier eating habits.

Increased Self-Efficacy: Engaging in regular exercise can boost self-efficacy, or the belief in one's ability to achieve goals. When individuals feel confident in their ability to make positive lifestyle choices, they are more likely to resist cravings for unhealthy foods or behaviors.

Distraction and Time Management: Exercise provides a productive and enjoyable way to distract oneself from cravings. Whether it's going for a run, practicing yoga, or participating in a team sport, physical activity can occupy both the mind and body, making it easier to resist the urge to indulge in cravings. Additionally, scheduling regular exercise sessions can help individuals manage their time more effectively and reduce opportunities for indulging in unhealthy behaviors.

Improved Sleep Quality: Regular exercise is linked to improved sleep quality and duration. Adequate sleep is crucial for regulating appetite hormones and reducing cravings. When well-rested, individuals are less likely to experience intense cravings for unhealthy foods or substances as a result of fatigue or disrupted sleep patterns.

Enhanced Self-Control and Willpower: Engaging in regular exercise requires discipline and self-control, which can spill over into other areas of life, including managing cravings. As individuals become accustomed to exercising self-control during workouts, they may find it easier to resist cravings for unhealthy foods or behaviors in other contexts.

Overcoming Challenges And Staying On Track

Overcoming challenges and staying on track in the journey to fix cravings and hunger habits requires resilience, persistence, and a positive mindset. Here are some strategies to help you navigate setbacks, cultivate resilience, and celebrate victories along the way:

Dealing with Setbacks:
Understand that setbacks are a normal part of any journey towards change. Instead of dwelling on setbacks, focus on learning from them and using them as opportunities for growth.

Identify what triggered the setback and brainstorm strategies to avoid similar situations in the future.

Strategies for Getting Back on Track:
When faced with a setback, don't let it derail your progress. Revisit your goals and remind yourself of your motivations for making changes. Take small, manageable steps to get back on track, such as recommitting to healthier habits or seeking support from friends, family, or a professional.

Cultivating Resilience and Persistence:
Cultivate resilience by developing coping skills to help you bounce back from challenges. Practice self-care activities such as mindfulness, exercise, and relaxation techniques to manage stress and build emotional resilience. Stay focused on your long-term goals and maintain a positive attitude, even in the face of obstacles.

Celebrating Victories:
No matter how tiny, appreciate and celebrate your accomplishments.. Celebrate your victories, whether it's sticking to a healthy eating plan for a week, resisting temptation when dining out, or choosing a nutritious snack over a less healthy option. Celebrating milestones helps to reinforce positive behaviors and boosts motivation to continue making healthy choices.

Setting Realistic Expectations:

Be realistic about your goals and expectations. Understand that fixing cravings and hunger habits is a gradual process that takes time and effort. Set achievable goals and celebrate progress along the way, rather than expecting instant results.

Seeking Support:
Don't be afraid to reach out for support when needed. Surround yourself with friends, family, or a support group who can provide encouragement, accountability, and motivation. Share your successes and challenges with others who understand and can offer support and guidance.
Practicing Self-Compassion:

Be kind to yourself throughout the journey. Treat yourself with the same compassion and understanding that you would offer to a friend facing similar challenges. Accept that perfection is not realistic and embrace the ups and downs of the process with self-compassion and forgiveness.

Reflection Prompt

Are you mindful of the foods you choose to purchase, or do you often make impulsive decisions while shopping? How can you incorporate healthier choices into your grocery shopping routine?

Reflect on your current meal preparation habits: Do you typically plan and prep meals in advance, or do you tend to make spontaneous food choices throughout the week?

What are your long-term goals for improving your eating habits and managing cravings? How can you continue to make progress towards these goals while also enjoying the journey along the way?

When faced with challenges or obstacles, do you tend to give up easily or persevere in finding solutions? What are some strategies you can use to bounce back from setbacks and stay on track?

____

____

____

____

How do you stay motivated and committed to your goals, even when faced with challenges or setbacks?

____

____

____

____

restaurant menus and choosing options that align with your health goals? What are some strategies you can use to make smart choices when dining away from home?

____

____

____

____

____

What are some practices or habits you can cultivate to build resilience and persistence over time?

____

____

____

____

Action plan

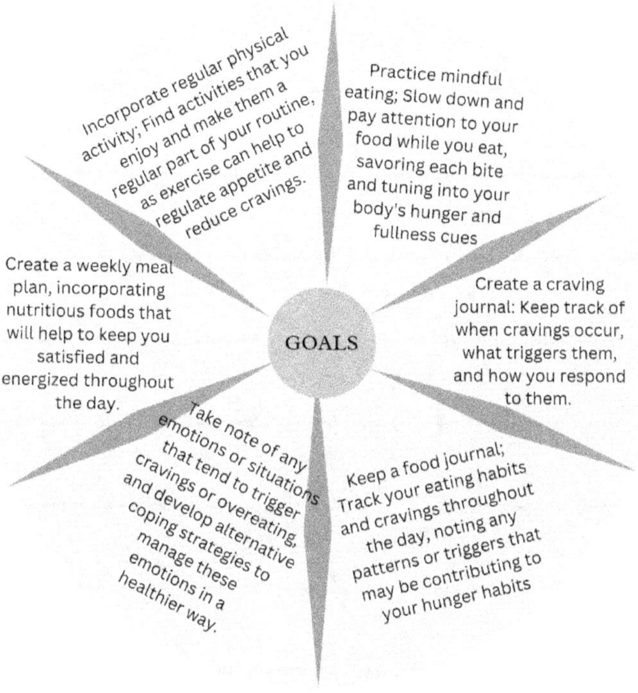

One step at a time let's go!

Journal your thoughts